A LITTLE BOOK OF DENTAL HYGIENISTS' RULES

ESTHER M. WILKINS, R.D.H., D.M.D.
Department of Periodontology
Tufts University School of Dental Medicine
Boston, Massachusetts

With contributions by
PATRICIA A. COHEN, R.D.H., B.S.
Private Practice
Boston, Massachusetts

Philadelphia
HANLEY & BELFUS, INC.

Published by HANLEY & BELFUS, INC., Medical Publishers,
210 South 13th Street, Philadelphia, PA 19107.
(215) 546-7293; 800-962-1892.
Internet: http//www.hanleyandbelfus.com

A LITTLE BOOK OF DENTAL HYGIENISTS' RULES   ISBN 1-56053-265-3
© 1998 by Hanley & Belfus, Inc.

Library of Congress catalog card number 97-74423

Last digit is the print number: 9 8 7 6 5 4 3 2 1

DEDICATION

To all dental hygienists around the world
  those who have practiced,
  those who are practicing now, and
  those students who will be practicing soon.

PREFACE

Everyone needs rules. They are a way of life. They keep us on our toes. They help us follow necessary routines in our professional world. Rules can act as guidelines. They can help us be ethically adept in professional practice.

With dental hygiene practice techniques, rules can mean the difference between success of a procedure or premature failure. For example, how long will a pit and fissure sealant last if rules of isolation and management of the materials are not followed to the letter? When rules of courtesy and kindness are not followed, patients may look elsewhere for their oral health care and services.

Research changes the rules periodically. We look back and chuckle at the rules we used to follow a few years ago. We smile and think, "Did we really do THAT?" A basic rule of life is: always be ready for change.

This little book of rules is about dental hygienists' practice, patients, colleagues, and personal relations. You will probably read only a few rules at a time. That's fine. There is no rush. There is no plot and no mystery to unravel.

It is expected that some rules will revitalize or reinforce your own rules. In the back of the book there is a form with an address so that you may send in new rules for inclusion in the next edition.

We hope that the gems of wit, wisdom, and experiences gathered here will be entertaining and educational. We hope you will enjoy this book—maybe to ponder or reflect a little, maybe to learn a little, and maybe to laugh a little.

Dental hygiene as a profession, according to the latest rumors, is going to be around for a long, long time. So keep it fresh. Keep it fun. And most of all, don't keep it to yourself.

Esther Wilkins, R.D.H., D.M.D.

If you would like to suggest a rule for the next edition, please photocopy this page as many times as needed and submit to the publisher. For information about ordering bulk quantities of the book for educational purposes, contact the publisher at 215-546-7293, or fax 215-790-9330.

Dental Hygienists' Rules
c/o Hanley & Belfus, Inc.
210 South 13th Street
Philadelphia, PA 19107

Rule: _____

_____

_____

_____

_____

_____

From (name and address): _____

_____

_____

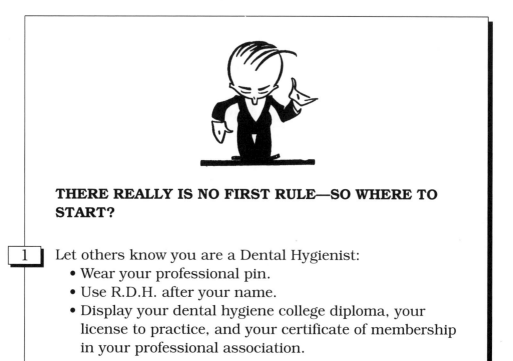

THERE REALLY IS NO FIRST RULE—SO WHERE TO START?

1 Let others know you are a Dental Hygienist:
   • Wear your professional pin.
   • Use R.D.H. after your name.
   • Display your dental hygiene college diploma, your license to practice, and your certificate of membership in your professional association.

| 2 | Honesty and integrity are the most important characteristics of a professional person. |

| 3 | The patient's welfare always comes first. |

| 4 | When patients say they cannot afford dentistry, help them understand how to afford prevention. |

| 5 | Think dental hygiene process:
- Assessment (Data Collection and Recording)
- Dental Hygiene Diagnosis
- Outcome Forecast (Prognosis)
- Planning
- Implementation (Interventions)
- Evaluation |

6 Four-handed dental hygiene is the way to go. Everyone benefits—dentist, dental hygienist, and especially the patient.

7 Think of 4-handed dental hygiene as 2-headed and 2-hearted.

8 The key to successful treatment is an accurate diagnosis. The key to an accurate diagnosis is knowledge of symptoms and probable causes.

9 Work together with other team members to prepare and update a policy manual.

10 Help select the reading material for the reception area. Avoid magazines that contradict your health messages of tobacco cessation and sugar-free snacks.

11 We do not classify people, but rather the disorders that people have. For example, refer to the "individual with diabetes" not the "diabetic." Never say "I've got an alcoholic (or an arthritic, or a cleft palate) in my chair."

12 Keep meticulous records. Document everything you do for a patient LEGIBLY—and in ink for permanent records.

Keep little notes: grandchildren that get awards; teenagers off to college.

| 13 | It is unethical and discriminatory to refuse treatment because of race, color, creed, sex, national origin, or because an individual is HIV-1 seropositive or has AIDS. |

| 14 | All rules for the clinical dental hygienist start with infection control. |

| 15 | Universal Precautions mean just that—universal. |

| 16 | Treat all patients the same way, as if they are infectious. |

17 Run water fast through the tubings for the air-water syringe for 1–2 minutes before the first appointment and then for 30 seconds between appointments.

18 Obtain all of your immunizations. Update them as indicated. Encourage your entire team to do likewise.

19 Use disposables whenever possible.

20 Take good care of your hands (your work depends on them):
- Keep nails short so they can't cut a glove; use lots of lotion.
- Keep cuticles pushed back and healthy.

21 First put on your mask and protective eyewear, then wash your hands and don your gloves. Never touch your hair, face, or mask during patient treatment.

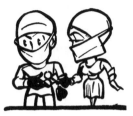

22 Wear your mask over your nose and mouth—not under your chin.

23 Never let a patient suck the saliva ejector.

24 Except for during treatment, sharpen instruments only when sterile and with a sterile sharpening stone.

25 Explain infection control materials and procedures so a patient will understand the steps taken to ensure complete safety.

26 Give patients a tour of the sterilization area.

27 Keep up to date on new exposure-control guidelines as well as new products on the market.

28 Greet each patient—even the last patient of a long day—with a warm smile and enthusiasm.

29 Never call a new patient over the age of 25 by the first name unless suggested by the patient. Show respect for all patients, especially senior citizens.

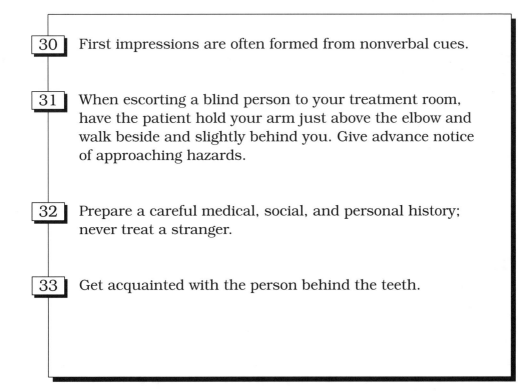

| 30 | First impressions are often formed from nonverbal cues. |

| 31 | When escorting a blind person to your treatment room, have the patient hold your arm just above the elbow and walk beside and slightly behind you. Give advance notice of approaching hazards. |

| 32 | Prepare a careful medical, social, and personal history; never treat a stranger. |

| 33 | Get acquainted with the person behind the teeth. |

| 34 | Make sure the patient speaks English before you get too far with long explanations. |

| 35 | Sit at eye level and look into the patient's eyes when you review the medical history. |

Inspire confidence.

| 36 | Show no reactions of approval or disapproval when preparing a history. |

| 37 | Speak clearly—don't mumble. |

When you are wearing a mask—speak louder.

| 38 | When the patient wants to talk, don't pretend you are listening—really listen. |

39 Include questions about allergies in the medical history—
especially latex allergy.
- Children can be allergic to latex. People with spina
  bifida are particularly sensitive to it.
- Latex allergens may lurk in rubber dam, prophy cups,
  orthodontic rings, nitrous oxide nosepieces, stoppers
  in anesthetic carpules, and many other products
  besides gloves.
- The only real protection against latex allergic
  reactions is to avoid the use of latex products.

40 When a patient cannot remember the
names of all current prescriptions,
ask to have the containers brought
in so you can study the possible
adaptations needed during dental
and dental hygiene appointments.

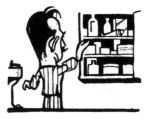

41 Keep up with current FDA approvals. Every year there are new products and new drugs. Check for possible side effects.

42 Measure and record vital signs.

43 Patients with a history of high blood pressure need to have it measured at each appointment; check every patient's blood pressure before administration of an anesthetic.

44 Encourage the patient on blood pressure medication to take the medication on schedule without fail.

45 Make a note in the appointment book when a patient requires antibiotic prophylaxis; remind the patient when confirming the appointment.

46 When a patient has not taken necessary premedication according to schedule, make a new appointment or only perform services that do not create a bacteremia.

47 Patients most likely to miss (or be late for) appointments are:
- those who do not receive a reminder (a day before phone call is better than mail)
- those who harbor fear of all dental treatments, and
- those who do not pay their own bills for dental health services.

48 List what you see as the attributes of a happy, satisfied patient. Then do and say things that will make patients happy and satisfied.

A DENTAL HYGIENIST'S WISH LIST

(in no particular order)

Patients who:

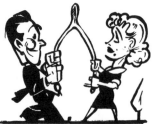

- arrive on time for appointments
- like to visit the dental hygienist
- brush and floss and then don't eat on the way to the appointment
- do not complain
- do not have to make a phone call and tie up the office phone
- are interested—and are interesting
- are compliant (floss every day for one thing)
- tell the truth and all the necessary facts with the medical history
- believe in me so much they refer others to me.

WISH LIST *(Continued)*

Long appointments, or at least long enough

Patients that do not use onions, garlic, tobacco, alcohol (or other offensive substances) 24 hours (at least) before their appointments

A really powerful saliva ejector

A quiet ultrasonic that doesn't shower aerosols over everything

Manual instruments that stay sharp

An ergonomically designed dental chair for the patient and clinic stool for the dental hygienist

A full-time assistant dedicated to dental hygiene

Anesthesia at a moment's notice (a wish from those not practicing where the law permits dental hygienists to administer local anesthesia)

An understanding and supportive colleague-dentist who believes 100% in the significance of what dental hygienists do.

| 50 | Perform an extraoral examination on every patient.

Enlarged lymph nodes can mean one of several things. |

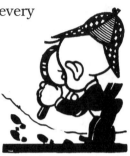

| 51 | What we see is what we look for— what we look for is what we know. |

| 52 | Remember that control and prevention of oral cancer depend on a thorough extraoral and intraoral examination for each patient at each visit. |

| 53 | Teach your patients the *Warning Signs of Oral Cancer* listed by one of the cancer societies. |

54 When a person is referred elsewhere for a biopsy, follow up to verify that the appointment was kept.

55 Check for oral evidence of physical abuse when a child presents with facial bruises or lacerations. Radiograph for jaw fracture; look for evidence of scarring from previous trauma.

56 You are a mandated reporter of abuse. Keep the phone number handy.

57 Probe every patient of every age.

58 First show the probe and explain what the marks mean. Demonstrate how an automated probe works if you use one.

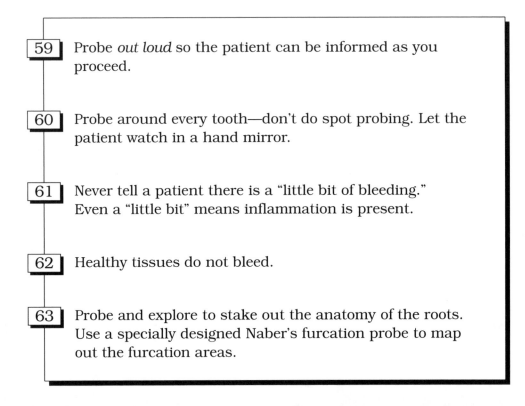

59 Probe *out loud* so the patient can be informed as you proceed.

60 Probe around every tooth—don't do spot probing. Let the patient watch in a hand mirror.

61 Never tell a patient there is a "little bit of bleeding." Even a "little bit" means inflammation is present.

62 Healthy tissues do not bleed.

63 Probe and explore to stake out the anatomy of the roots. Use a specially designed Naber's furcation probe to map out the furcation areas.

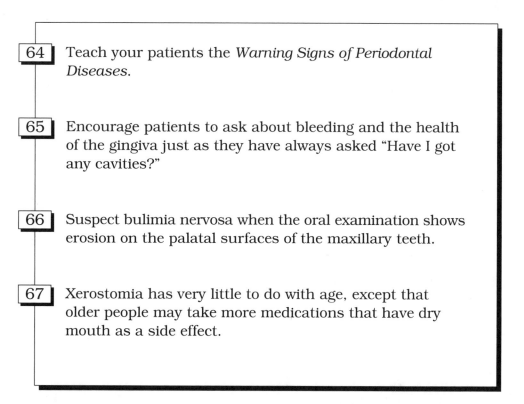

64 Teach your patients the *Warning Signs of Periodontal Diseases*.

65 Encourage patients to ask about bleeding and the health of the gingiva just as they have always asked "Have I got any cavities?"

66 Suspect bulimia nervosa when the oral examination shows erosion on the palatal surfaces of the maxillary teeth.

67 Xerostomia has very little to do with age, except that older people may take more medications that have dry mouth as a side effect.

68 When you explore for dental caries, include checking around the sealants; then schedule repairs or replacements when needed.

69 Expect a sealant to last at least 15 years when careful, precise placement procedures are followed.

70 When a patient asks about the dangers of dental x-ray exposure, explain the safety features, including fast film, insulated equipment, and the lead apron with the thyroid collar.

71 Perfect your radiographic techniques so you rarely need a retake.

72 Set up the patient care plan using the assessment data collected and the patient's risk factors.

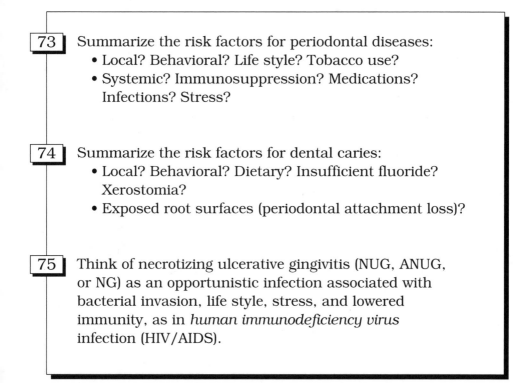

73 Summarize the risk factors for periodontal diseases:
- Local? Behavioral? Life style? Tobacco use?
- Systemic? Immunosuppression? Medications? Infections? Stress?

74 Summarize the risk factors for dental caries:
- Local? Behavioral? Dietary? Insufficient fluoride? Xerostomia?
- Exposed root surfaces (periodontal attachment loss)?

75 Think of necrotizing ulcerative gingivitis (NUG, ANUG, or NG) as an opportunistic infection associated with bacterial invasion, life style, stress, and lowered immunity, as in *human immunodeficiency virus* infection (HIV/AIDS).

76 NUG is an AIDS-indicator disease. Oral manifestations may be the first signs of HIV-1 infection.

77 About 50% of American children between the ages 7 and 17 currently have no cavities and never did. That's fine—but the important fact to know for dental hygienists is that 50% DO have dental caries.

78 Promote prevention and control of dental caries by placing more sealants.

79 Show patients with xerostomia how to use daily 5-minute applications of 1.1% sodium fluoride (neutral) in a custom-fitted tray.

80 Do not use acidulated fluoride for patients with porcelain or composite restorations.

81   Advise sugar-free gum, mints, etc. for people with xerostomia, or anyone with a dental caries problem (for those that use them).

82   Practice anticipatory guidance—teach before it happens.

83   Teach parents to maintain their own oral health so they cannot pass *Mutans streptococci* and other microorganisms to their babies.

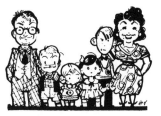

84   Also teach them to use only water if a baby/nursing bottle is given at bed or nap time. Cariogenic bacteria multiply fast in a baby's mouth if cariogenic substances are available often.

85 | Be aware that anticipatory guidance applies to people of all ages. For instance, help elderly people to follow caries prevention methods for root caries.

86 | Promote periodontal health during pregnancy. A mother-to-be with periodontal infection has more than 7 times the risk of having a baby with preterm low birth rate (compared with mothers with no periodontal infection).

87 | **SOME CHAIRSIDE RULES**
- If your patient asks a question and you do not know the answer, say you do not know, but you will find out.
- Keep secrets—it's professional.
- Leave office information in the office; respect confidentiality.

- Never discuss patients within earshot of other patients.
- Do not take telephone calls during a dental hygiene appointment. Tell your friends and family to call you at home.
- When you try out a new procedure, never reveal that it is the first time you've done it.
- Do not do unto others anything you would not want others to do unto you.
- Always exude confidence in front of a patient—but modesty is still the best policy.
- Skip the perfume—your patient may be allergic to it or annoyed by it.
- Forget about selling tickets to a patient—even for your favorite charity event.
- Never discuss your personal life with a patient.
- Put things back where they belong.

88 Without a "care plan" or treatment plan, you cannot know where you are going, so you'll probably end up somewhere else, and not know where you are.

89 When the care plan is reviewed with the patient, do not hesitate to tell a patient how severe the oral condition or problem really is. That way the patient will be more likely to understand the number of appointments needed and the responsibility of daily self-care.

90 For the periodontal aspects of your instrumentation, never tell a patient you will "clean" the teeth. Let the patient do the cleaning with toothbrush and floss—at home in the bathroom. *You* do preventive or curative therapy.

91 Explain the need for quadrant treatment with anesthesia and what you expect to accomplish.

92 Make use of the quadrant appointment plan to help your patients climb further up the Learning Ladder: From

Unaware—to Aware—to Self-interest—to Belief— to Commitment—to **ACTION!**

By that time they really will have a great plaque-free score.

93 Anticipate the endpoints of therapy: reduced signs of infection and inflammation, especially no bleeding on probing, and reduced probing depths.

| 94 | Tell your patient what the immediate goals are, and that after this part of the treatment you will reevaluate and set new goals. |

| 95 | Do not promise complete cure. Control of periodontal infections takes daily bacterial plaque removal throughout life. |

| 96 | Start with instruction. *Inform before you Perform.* |

| 97 | First, have the patient learn basic bacterial control (floss and brush) to prepare a clean mouth before you scale. It is a tissue conditioning process. |

98 There will be fewer contaminated aerosols (to get into your hair and on the uncovered parts of your face) when the mouth is brushed and flossed prior to instrumentation.

99 Preprocedural antibacterial rinsing is routine for dental as well as dental hygiene services. Chlorhexidine rinses still have the most substantivity.

100 Preprocedural rinsing reduces contamination in the aerosols but does even better in terms of lowering the bacteremias created.

101 Scoop that needle cover! Never re-cap directly.

102 If you practice where you cannot give the injection of anesthetic yourself, help the dentist by noting on the daily schedule what time you will need anesthesia. That way it is on her or his mind and is not really an interruption.

103 Check the blood pressure and the medical history before selecting the anesthetic. Certain patients should not be given epinephrine, such as when you suspect cocaine use.

104 Decrease eye strain and improve the quality of your instrumentation by using vision scopes. Optimal eye-to-object working distance facilitates good posture.

105 Practice good posture. Sit on the entire seat, not on the edge.

106 Arrange and adapt the dental hygiene treatment area to the comfort and needs of you, the clinician. The patient will be there a relatively short time.

107 Cumulative trauma affects not only your hands. Move around and do "stretchies" for your shoulders and back regularly throughout the day. Remember: the hand bones are connected to the arm bones, the arm bones are connected to the shoulder bones, the shoulder bones are connected to the back bones, the back bones are connected to the neck bones . . .

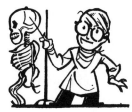

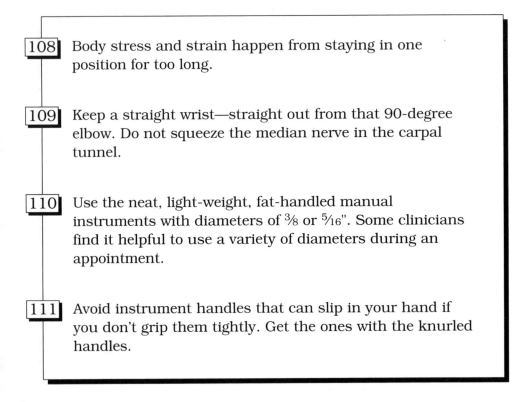

|108| Body stress and strain happen from staying in one position for too long.

|109| Keep a straight wrist—straight out from that 90-degree elbow. Do not squeeze the median nerve in the carpal tunnel.

|110| Use the neat, light-weight, fat-handled manual instruments with diameters of $\frac{3}{8}$ or $\frac{5}{16}$". Some clinicians find it helpful to use a variety of diameters during an appointment.

|111| Avoid instrument handles that can slip in your hand if you don't grip them tightly. Get the ones with the knurled handles.

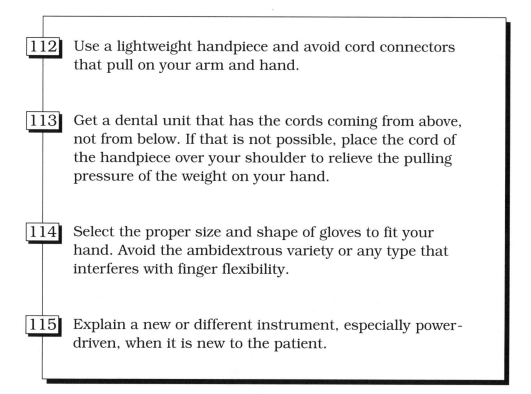

112 Use a lightweight handpiece and avoid cord connectors that pull on your arm and hand.

113 Get a dental unit that has the cords coming from above, not from below. If that is not possible, place the cord of the handpiece over your shoulder to relieve the pulling pressure of the weight on your hand.

114 Select the proper size and shape of gloves to fit your hand. Avoid the ambidextrous variety or any type that interferes with finger flexibility.

115 Explain a new or different instrument, especially power-driven, when it is new to the patient.

116 Do minimal scaling in shallow pockets (it can lead to loss of attachment) but, of course, be sure the surface is smooth.

117 Your instrument is an extension of yourself. Go gently into those deep dark pockets but be thorough in the deposit removal.

118 Excellence is a habit.

119 Maintain the correct working angle at the cutting edge of scalers and curets. Angles below 65 degrees and above 85 degrees will be less functional.

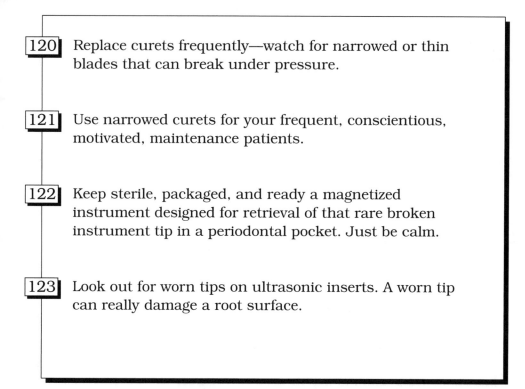

120 Replace curets frequently—watch for narrowed or thin blades that can break under pressure.

121 Use narrowed curets for your frequent, conscientious, motivated, maintenance patients.

122 Keep sterile, packaged, and ready a magnetized instrument designed for retrieval of that rare broken instrument tip in a periodontal pocket. Just be calm.

123 Look out for worn tips on ultrasonic inserts. A worn tip can really damage a root surface.

124 Ultrasonic tips do not last forever. Check them every New Year's Day.

125 Use of an ultrasonic scaler has been shown to produce almost 3 times more contaminated aerosols per unit of air sampled than manual instruments—another reason for preprocedural toothbrushing as well as antibacterial rinsing.

126 Practice principles of selective stain removal. If there is no stain, do not polish. You know—if it ain't broke, don't fix it.

127 Do not open up the dentinal tubules at cervical areas by overdoing your rubber cup with a too-abrasive polishing paste. The teeth can become very sensitive.

128 If you want patients to really love you, treat sensitive cervical areas by applying a desensitizing agent. Recommend a fluoride dentrifice for home use that contains a desensitizer such as potassium nitrate.

129 Reshape and polish overhangs or chart them for replacement.

130 Watch for young (and old) active sports patients—make a mouthguard if they do not have one.

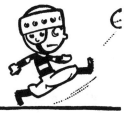

131 Develop partnerships with your patients—you do your part and they do their part.

| 132 | Learn to give health risk messages that will motivate good behaviors and prevent harmful outcomes. |

| 133 | When a patient says "No one ever told me that before," SMILE! Seize the opportunity to raise the Dental and Periodontal IQs even higher. |

| 134 | An ounce of oral disease prevention is worth a pound of cure. |

| 135 | Do not talk over the patient's head using technical terms. |

| 136 | Compliment patients who try hard. |

137 An apple a day keeps the dentist away—when it is eaten instead of a cariogenic food or sweet.

138 Never assume that just because a patient has worn dentures for years that he or she knows how to clean them.

139 Be sure to make it real clear what "plaque" is in the mouth. Some people hang plaques on the wall—their diplomas and awards.

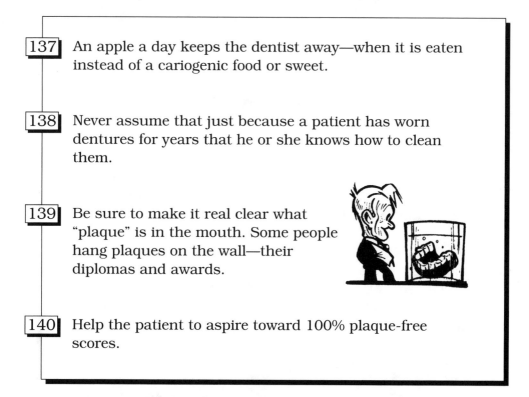

140 Help the patient to aspire toward 100% plaque-free scores.

141 Use a disclosing agent and a mirror to show and tell.

142 Watch to see that the patient curves the floss into a "C" to clean all sides and angles of each tooth.

143 Have the patient thread new floss into a floss threader right after using. Then hang the floss with threader over the toothbrush so it is always ready for the next time.

144 Challenge the patient to see how long the floss threader can be used. Floss threaders have been known to last into the second year and then be lost only because the patient carried it on a camping trip.

|145| It is not the brush: it is the hand that holds it and the head that tells the hand what to do that determine how much bacterial plaque will be cleaned off.

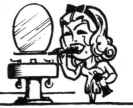

|146| Never give out a toothbrush without a lesson. Preferably give the brush only after the patient has practiced correct brushing in the mouth.

|147| Offer advice and recommendations about power-driven toothbrushes, including the advantages of some of the approved ones on the market.

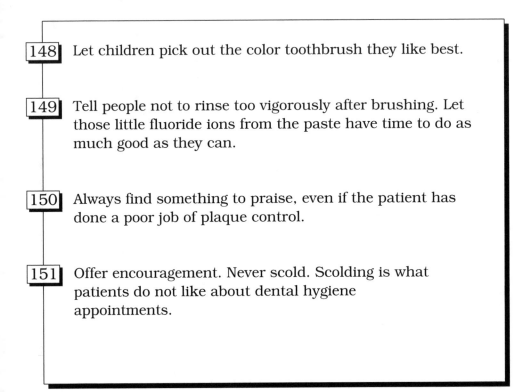

148 Let children pick out the color toothbrush they like best.

149 Tell people not to rinse too vigorously after brushing. Let those little fluoride ions from the paste have time to do as much good as they can.

150 Always find something to praise, even if the patient has done a poor job of plaque control.

151 Offer encouragement. Never scold. Scolding is what patients do not like about dental hygiene appointments.

152 Never say "Remember what I told you at our last appointment?" Just patiently start over with a different approach.

153 When a patient believes everything will be okay as long as the appointments with you are kept faithfully, start back at step one. Explain again about the bacteria that live on and around each tooth and how they multiply <u>every day</u>.

154 Do not threaten that the teeth will be lost. The patient may have grandparents who apparently get along fine with the complete dentures they have had for 40 years.

155 Say goodbye to that old paradigm that everyone will lose teeth eventually and need dentures. Also say goodbye to other sayings, such as:
- Why save the baby teeth—they are going to fall out anyway.
- Dental caries is a disease of children; gum disease is in old people.
- Milk is for babies.

156 Fluoride is not just for kids. Everyone benefits from fluoride.

157 Drink fluoridated water every day—and use it to make the baby's formula and to make soup.

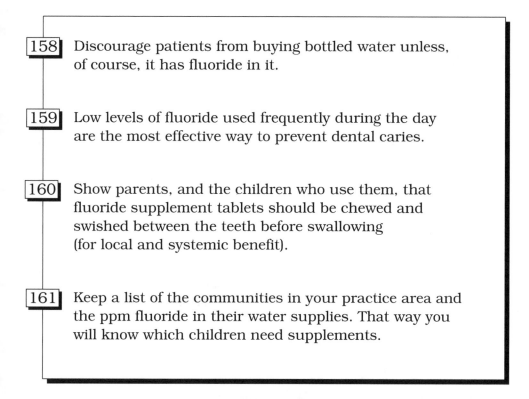

158 Discourage patients from buying bottled water unless, of course, it has fluoride in it.

159 Low levels of fluoride used frequently during the day are the most effective way to prevent dental caries.

160 Show parents, and the children who use them, that fluoride supplement tablets should be chewed and swished between the teeth before swallowing (for local and systemic benefit).

161 Keep a list of the communities in your practice area and the ppm fluoride in their water supplies. That way you will know which children need supplements.

162 Assist families with private water sources to have the water tested for fluoride content before the dentist, pediatric dentist, or pediatrician prescribes supplements.

163 Professional topical fluoride applications are still important, particularly for caries-susceptible patients. Include among those the patients with xerostomia and junk-food-eating teenagers and adults.

164 Do not overfill the fluoride gel tray for children. Two milliliters is enough for small children and 2.5 ml for larger patients. Measure it once and see where it comes in the tray. After that you can estimate the amount.

165 Visit the exhibits at dental meetings to learn about new products.

166 Try all the samples (brushes, floss, interdental devices, tongue cleaners, and so forth) so you can speak from experience when patients ask about a product they saw advertised.

167 Visit the oral hygiene section of stores in the neighborhood of your practice.
- Know where patients can purchase devices and products you want them to use.
- Ask the store owner to carry the products you recommend.

168 Read the research literature so you can evaluate manufacturers' claims.

169 Hold on to things that work.

170 Write letters to your voting governmental officials to indicate your stand on a particular public health issue.

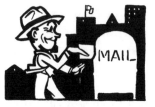

171 For the terminally ill person, comfort is of more value than restorative treatment. Help provide daily cleansing to give the mouth a comfortable clean feeling and a nice taste.

|172| If a patient swallows an object during an appointment, get prompt medical care and x-ray to locate the object.

Do not take chances on whether it is in a lung or the alimentary tract.

|173| Another reason for 4-handed dental hygiene is that the assistant can grab the high-volume suction should an object go into the oropharynx.

|174| Be aware of the universal sign of airway obstruction: the person is grasping the throat with a frantic look on the face and cannot speak.

|175| The first 6 minutes are the most crucial. Give oxygen for a patient who is breathing but partially obstructed.

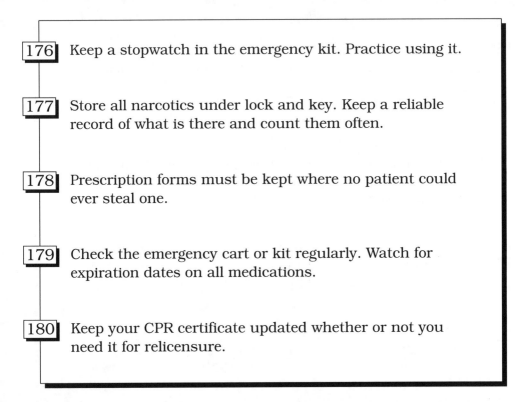

176   Keep a stopwatch in the emergency kit. Practice using it.

177   Store all narcotics under lock and key. Keep a reliable record of what is there and count them often.

178   Prescription forms must be kept where no patient could ever steal one.

179   Check the emergency cart or kit regularly. Watch for expiration dates on all medications.

180   Keep your CPR certificate updated whether or not you need it for relicensure.

181 Nitroglycerin under the tongue of a patient with xerostomia will not dissolve.

Add a few drops of water.

182 When a patient refuses to have radiographs or some type of essential treatment, get a signed statement.

183 It is important to inform an individual of the risks of non-treatment.

184 Include smoking status as a new vital sign, and record it along with blood pressure, pulse, respiration, and body temperature. Smoking is the most preventable cause of death.

185 Place specific questions regarding tobacco use on the medical history form.

186 For the patient who uses tobacco, have a Tobacco-use Assessment Form ready to obtain complete information.

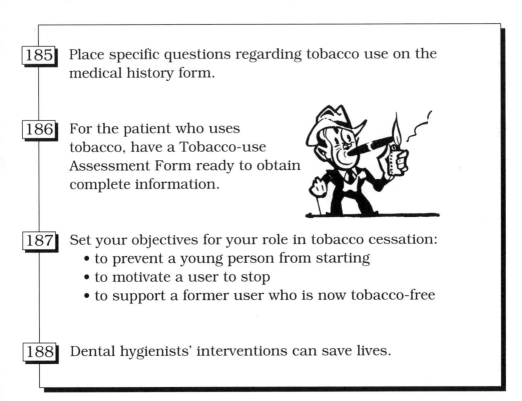

187 Set your objectives for your role in tobacco cessation:
- to prevent a young person from starting
- to motivate a user to stop
- to support a former user who is now tobacco-free

188 Dental hygienists' interventions can save lives.

189 Learn techniques to assist the patient in tobacco cessation:
- Take a continuing education course
- Obtain materials from the National Cancer Institute

190 Learn and use a brief intervention message to help your patients quit using tobacco. When they are ready, help to provide tobacco cessation counseling.

191 Inform patients that tobacco use is a major risk factor for periodontal diseases and oral cancer.

192 Help patients understand the adverse effects of tobacco use on the bone and soft tissue around the teeth. It also slows the healing process.

193 When implants are being considered, smoking habits should be on the list of contraindications.

More implants fail in smokers than in nonsmokers.

194 Obtain team cooperation to make your practice setting smoke-free.

Display "Thank You for Not Smoking" signs and remove ashtrays.

195 Add tobacco education information to the anticipatory guidance for patients. Include information about the effect of environmental second-hand smoke during pregnancy as well as on people in the household.

196 Learning never ends. Select continuing education courses to keep you informed about new scientific developments and trends in dental hygiene practice.

197 Enjoy continuing education courses for their own sake—not only because they help to renew your license.

198 When you relocate, check the laws, rules, and regulations of your new state or province.

199 The dental hygienist is accountable legally and ethically for the quality of dental hygiene services performed.

200 Be an active member of local, state, national, and international dental hygienists' associations and enjoy the benefits.

201 No man is an island—make friends with other dental hygienists at the meetings.

202 Read your association newsletters and journals. Write a letter to the editor when something pleases or concerns you.

203 Keep an open mind—there is a lot of new research out there, and more on the way.

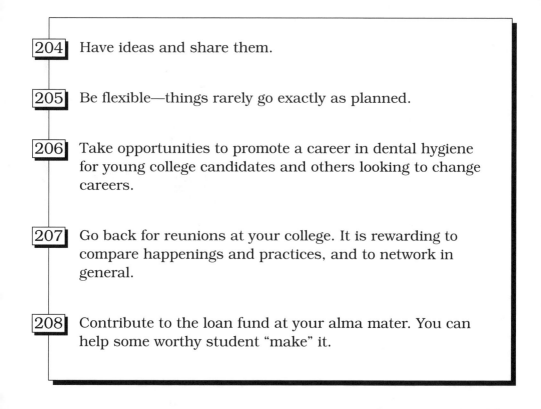

|204| Have ideas and share them.

|205| Be flexible—things rarely go exactly as planned.

|206| Take opportunities to promote a career in dental hygiene for young college candidates and others looking to change careers.

|207| Go back for reunions at your college. It is rewarding to compare happenings and practices, and to network in general.

|208| Contribute to the loan fund at your alma mater. You can help some worthy student "make" it.

WHAT TO DO WHEN YOU THINK BURN-OUT IS IMMINENT

Start by writing down a list of everything that is **bad** about your situation. <u>Underline</u> those that can be changed.

Make a list of everything that is **good** about your situation. <u>Underline</u> the most valuable.

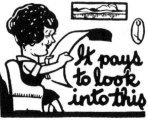

- Reread letters from your grateful patients.
- Picture your most rewarding patient experiences.
- Think of your favorite patients and why they are your favorites.

Evaluate your lists and make an Action Plan.

Your Action Plan may include:

- Join or form a study club.
- Join a book club.

- Volunteer: the heart association? library? science museum?
- Help prepare and serve meals at a local shelter; deliver meals on wheels to homebound people.

Seek out a **mentor** for inspiration and advice.

Matriculate for credit courses toward your next higher degree.

Make appointments for a facial or a complete professional body massage for each week for the next 10 weeks.

Order new sets of curets with all the new styles and forms.

Try new things: products, instruments, and more.

Get involved in a community effort to get fluoride in the drinking water.

Change your practice routine over to do 4-handed
dental hygiene.
- Hire and train an assistant.
- Show your colleague-dentist how your dental
  hygiene department can increase income by more
  than the salary of the assistant.

Get more active in your dental hygiene associations.
Volunteer for office and aim to become a delegate
to the national meeting.

Take a nice long vacation.

Plan the vacation so you can attend the IFDH
(International Federation of Dental Hygienists) and
meet dental hygienists from around the world.

210 Laugh and enjoy life: people like people who enjoy their
work and show it.

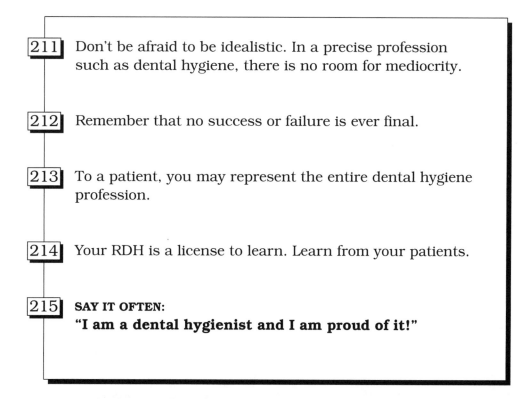

|211| Don't be afraid to be idealistic. In a precise profession such as dental hygiene, there is no room for mediocrity.

|212| Remember that no success or failure is ever final.

|213| To a patient, you may represent the entire dental hygiene profession.

|214| Your RDH is a license to learn. Learn from your patients.

|215| **SAY IT OFTEN:**
"I am a dental hygienist and I am proud of it!"

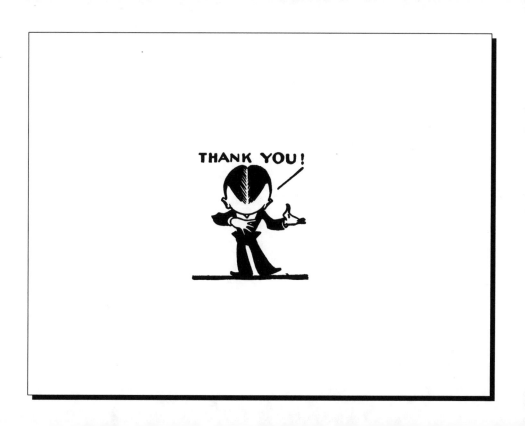

If you would like to suggest a rule for the next edition, please photocopy this page as many times as needed and submit to the publisher. For information about ordering bulk quantities of the book for educational purposes, contact the publisher at 215-546-7293, or fax 215-790-9330.

Dental Hygienists' Rules
c/o Hanley & Belfus, Inc.
210 South 13th Street
Philadelphia, PA 19107

Rule: _____

_____

_____

_____

_____

_____

_____

From (name and address): _____

_____

_____